INTERMITTENT FASTING MEAL PLAN

GET LEAN AND RIPPED FAST!

From Anthony Cooke

Cover designed by Anthony Cooke
Written by Anthony Cooke
Edited by Joymemo
Published by Amazon Create Space

CONTENTS

One

Positive Comments from the YouTube Community

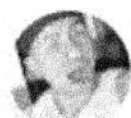

Ray 8 months ago

This works I do the 16/8 I was 200 pounds 3 months ago started IF now I'm down to 170 with my abs showing I have 3 meals a day I eat about 2,200 cal a day and only workout 3 days a week for only 1hr

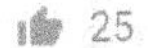 25   REPLY

View 3 replies ˅

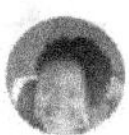

jenngjones24 1 year ago

Thanks so much. This was easy to understand and easy to follow. I will be starting my 16/8 lifestyle over. I'm excited...again!

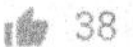 38  REPLY

ksfs09 1 year ago (edited)

Finally a clear video on exactly what to eat on IF!. Thank you!. Also and most importantly I like that you're not forgetting about your overall health and adding the vegetable juice. I do have a question. Can you drink your vegetable juice any time during your intermittent fasting window? or does it have to be with your meal?

 90   REPLY

Hide replies ˄

 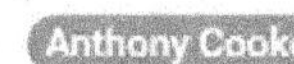 **Anthony Cooke** 1 year ago

ksfs09 You can drink it anytime during your eating window it doesn't have to be with a meal. You don't want to drink it in your fasting window though because it does have calories.

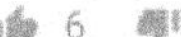 6  REPLY

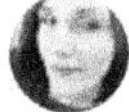

Racheli Snovsky 1 year ago

wow!!! those are awesome meals!!! very nutrition dense! I'm new to intermittent fasting and have a lot to learn.. thanks for sharing what works for you!

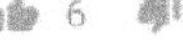 2  REPLY

Hide replies ˄

 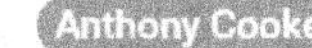 **Anthony Cooke** 1 year ago

You're Welcome!

  REPLY

1

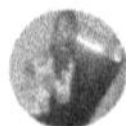
hunnyb1308 1 year ago

Thank you Anthony for this very clear, and informative video. I've been searching for a video like this. I started IF kinda accidentally. However, I realized for several weeks, that I was losing inches, and a couple pounds.

Read more

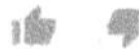 REPLY

Hide replies ∧

 **Anthony Cooke** 1 year ago

hunnyb1308 You're Welcome

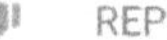 REPLY

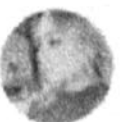
Marta XO 1 year ago (edited)

Apparently, with IF, it's best to exercise on an empty stomach before your first meal. Your meals look delicious, btw!

 REPLY

Hide replies ∧

 **Anthony Cooke** 1 year ago

Thank You! In my experience I've tried both, and haven't noticed much difference as far as fat loss / muscle gains go. The biggest difference that I have noticed though is 'energy'. If I have a meal before I workout I will have much more energy for my workouts.

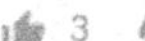 3  REPLY

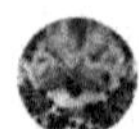
Raging Fury 16 hours ago

100% agree, IF was what got me to lose my weight, I work in Saudi Arabia and it's just too damn hot during the summer to do IF so usually for 6 months I'll do IF and during the summer ill just take it slow lol.

 REPLY

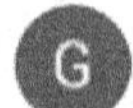
Gs5v5 7bv6tv 8 months ago

Thank you for a clear video about IF, this has been the best video I've seen about it and it helped a lot thank you !

 REPLY

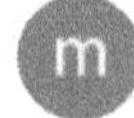
marco polo 7 months ago

Excellent video brotha! Thanks for showing us the simple diet plan! Awesome!it's healthy and it's simple to follow, thanks

 REPLY

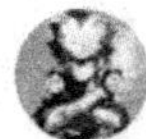
Mobstar Hipstar 1 year ago

wow finally IF done high in vegetables

 15   REPLY

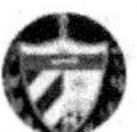
Marcos Garcia 1 week ago

Thank you bro, I've been at it for a week now, and it's been real easy for despite being over weight and 42 years old.. Been easy so far. Thanks again bud..

  REPLY

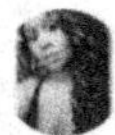
findjoselyn 2 months ago

Mannnn, this is AWESOME! I love how you explained everything and provided your macros.

  REPLY

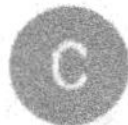
CanoJR 1 year ago

Thanks for the video! I've been IF for 1.5 months now and I'm down 36 lbs and 5 inches off my waist. I tweaked some of your recipes a bit and found out what works for me. IF is the real deal!

   REPLY

Hide replies ^

  1 year ago

CanoJR You're Welcome. That is awesome!

  REPLY

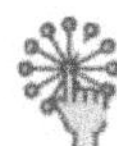
Max Bianco 4 months ago

Thanks for this info man. Appreciate you. I hope it works out for me as well.

  REPLY

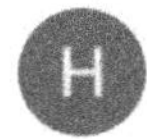
Harry Maynard 7 months ago

I can't believe how quick my six pack actually came in 😁

  REPLY

My Progress after 7 Weeks of this Intermittent Fasting Meal Plan

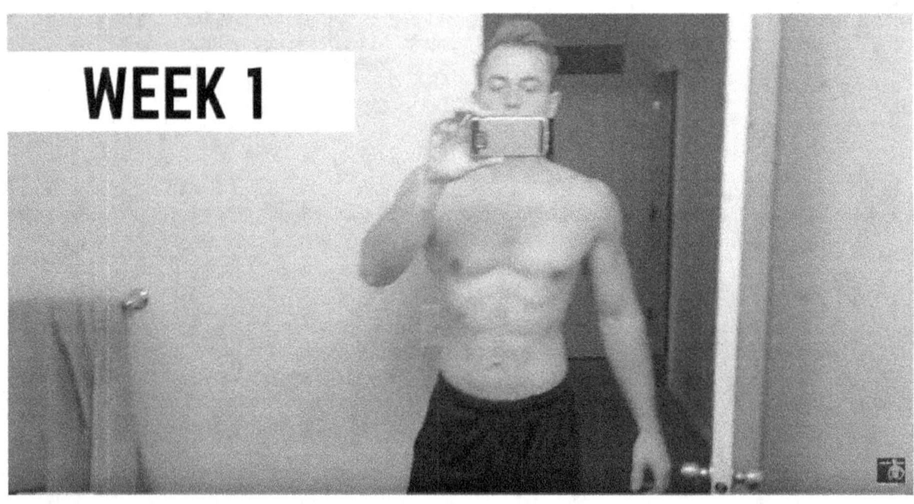

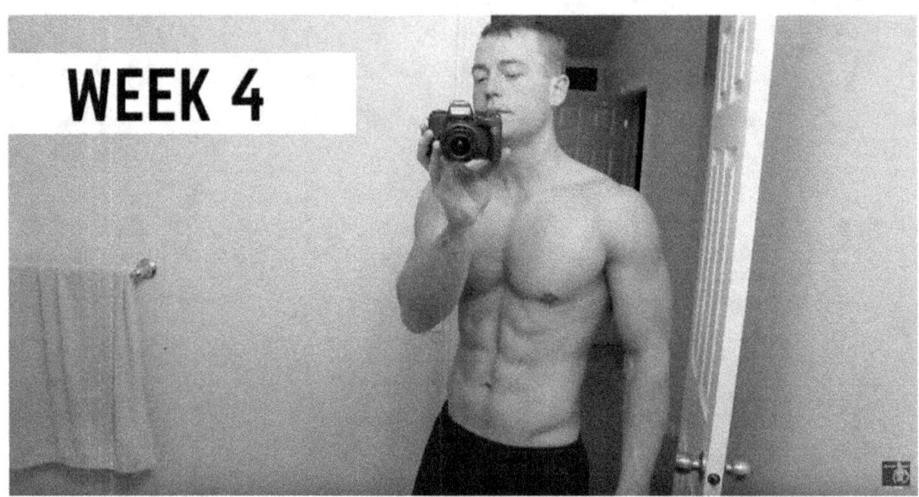

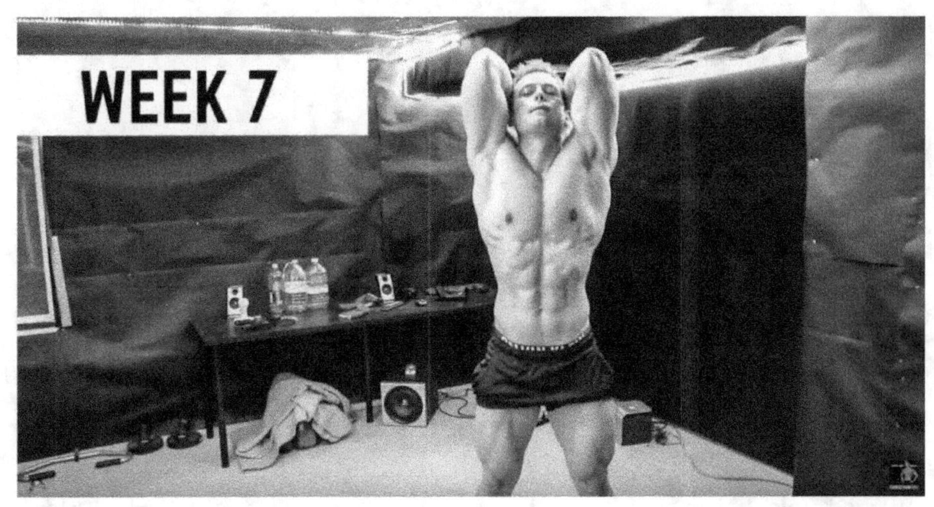

YouTube Channel:https://bit.ly/2oPdUI9

Instagram: https://www.instagram.com/anthonylcooke/

SnapChat: ALC4

Three

Introduction to Intermittent Fasting Meal Plan get Lean and Ripped Fast!

In this book, I share with you my exact intermittent fasting meal plan to get lean and ripped. I have been putting intermittent fasting into practice for some years now, and it has always helped me burn fat very well. When I first found intermittent fasting, it was in an attempt to find out how I could burn the fat that had been in my body forever and finally reveal my six pack abs. I came across a very well-known method that is used heavily today, 16 8. This means that you fast for 16 hours and have an 8-hour eating window to consume all your food in a 24hour day. This is the exact intermittent fasting method that I still used today, with a slight variation.

After experiencing and studying intermittent fasting for many years, I would have to say that the reason it works so well is that it increases your growth hormone. The main hormone in your body that is responsible for burning fat. This is where my slight variation comes into play. With that being the key, I only eat two meals a day. This gives me the best combination to keep my growth hormone high and my insulin levels low so that I can burn the most amount of fat possible while staying full all day long.

According to Dr. Berg an extremely qualified individual on nutrition science and who has taught as an associate professor at Howard University says, "Every time we eat, our insulin levels spike shutting off our fat burning hormone which is the growth hormone." This is why like many professional doctors I believe that intermittent fasting and only having two meals a day is a great way to keep your growth hormone high and insulin levels low so that you can burn the most amount of fat possible.

If you read and follow through this entire book, which I hope you will do, there are going to be a few key points that are very important to watch for. You will notice that the main staple of my intermittent fasting meal plan is greens. The reason why greens are so good and necessary is that they are loaded with micronutrients, vitamins, and minerals. They help you stay full all day long. They are low in calories, which is very important for losing weight because being in a calorie deficit is necessary if you want to lose weight. Also because of the micronutrients, you will notice that your body functions a lot better and you will even see your outward appearance change like having clearer skin.

Put this intermittent fasting meal plan into practice and watch the magic unfold. You don't necessarily have to eat what I have shown in this book. The main things you need to eat are lots of greens, a few fruits, and proteins. Keep away from sugar, processed food, bread, and pasta. These types of food will spike your insulin thereby shutting off fat burning.

Four

What to do While Fasting

While intermittent fasting, you'll be running off an eating window and a fasting window. What I want to address in this section is what to do during your fasting window. The window of time where you will be consuming ZERO CALORIES! That means no food that contains calories is being consumed.

I will mention a few key things here if it's your first-time intermittent fasting. Yes, you will get hungry. Yes, your mind will play tricks on you and tempt you to eat, but you are strong and will not fall for such trickery of the mind!

During your fasting window, you can consume anything that has zero calories, which boils down the list to water, and zero calorie drinks, such as black coffee, green tea, sparkling water, and zero calorie energy drinks.

The best strategy I have found that works, is keeping water at hand all the time. Just carry a gallon of water all day if you must or have some close by that you can access. Whatever your preference, drink plenty of water. It will help with the hunger slightly if that's an issue and of course keep you hydrated.

There are going to be times when the hunger gets unbearable while you're waiting for your first meal of the day. I have two options in this scenario. I will drink sparkling water which helps blunt hunger or either drink some black coffee since it has zero calories. I will note the drinks with caffeine that help blunt hunger the most. This will get you to your first meal of the day without having to deal with the pain of not eating for many hours.

Five

Working out While Intermittent Fasting

I want to address working out while intermittent fasting briefly. I have my eating window from 12 pm (noon) to 8 p.m. and then fast from 8 p.m. to 12 pm (noon) the next day. This brings up a ubiquitous question that I see often.

What if you work out in the morning?

The answer is, it doesn't matter when you work out. You can work out anytime you feel like. Just realize one thing; if you work out during your fasting window, you are likely going to have less energy than if you're working out during your eating window because you would most likely have had either your first meal of the day or a snack before your work out.

Choose whichever fits your schedule best. The results for working out while fasting vs. non-fasting are going to be the same regardless of what you choose as long as you're consistent.

Six

Liver Detox Shake

The liver detox shake is an essential part of this intermittent fasting meal plan that I picked up from Dr. Eric Berg who is a major influence on YouTube in the health niche with over 1,800,000 subscribers and his videos being viewed over 241,841,219 times. The benefits are endless; first, it provides cleansing for a fatty liver, this is very important because your liver is responsible for over 50000+ processes in your body. Having a clean liver will help you burn fat faster, and retain lean muscle mass better. Secondly, it provides you with massive amounts of potassium (natural energy) and essential vitamins and minerals. In addition to helping you become lean and ripped, this shake is going to give you a healthy glow, mental clarity and a lot of energy.

Directions: Drink this shake once a day either with meal one or meal two or anytime during your eating window.

Ingredients:

- 3 cups of frozen kale
- 1 cup of frozen beat tops (cut the tops of the beats off)
- 1 cup of frozen parsley
- 1 kiwi
- ½ cup blueberry
- ½ cup strawberry
- 3 drops of stevia

Instructions;

Place all ingredients in a blender, add enough water so that the blender can blend it into a nice liquid shake, add one cup of ice if desired and blend everything.

Seven

Breaking Your Fast, First Meal of the Day

The first meal of the day usually starts at noon or later for me, because I set my eating window from noon to 8 p.m as I mentioned earlier in section five.

The main bulk of the meal includes lots of leafy greens, substantial amounts of protein, healthy fats, and a few carbohydrates to top it off.

Main Course: Protein Salad

Ingredients:

- 2 to 4 handfuls of mixed leafy greens
- 3/4 pound of ground chicken
- 3 eggs
- A small handful of blueberry's
- A few mushrooms
- Walden farms zero calorie dressing

Side: Rice Cakes with Almond Butter

- 1 to 4 rice cakes
- 1 Tbsp. of almond butter on each rice cake

Drink: Lemon Water with Apple Cider Vinegar

- 8 oz of water
- 1 shot of apple cider vinegar
- 1 shot of lemon juice

Main Course Instructions;

First, find a large bowl and or container. Put 2 to 4 handfuls of leafy mixed greens in the bowl.

Cook one pound of ground chicken on the stove using medium to high heat until completely done. Add your favorite seasoning in small amounts as you cook. Once the chicken is completely cooked, add it to the bowl.

Next scramble or fry 1 to 3 eggs whichever you prefer in a saucepan by first spreading one tps of grass-fed butter or olive oil in the pan on a stove with medium to high heat, adding salt and pepper if you like and once completely done, add the eggs to the salad bowl.

Finally, add your toppings blueberries and mushrooms or other vegetables to the protein salad and drizzle on as much Walden farms zero calories dressing as you like.

Side Instructions;

On a plate place 1 to 4 rice cakes. For each rice cake, you spread one tbsp. of almond butter on it.

Drink Instructions;

Fill an 8-ounce glass 2/3 full of water. Add one shot of apple cider vinegar and one shot of lemon juice. Mix well and drink.

Estimate of Meal one

Calories: 1,074

Protein: 91g

Carbs: 61g

Fats 54g

Eight

Second Meal of the Day, Starting Your Fast Again

The second meal of the day for me is consumed about 30 minutes to an hour before my eating window closes. I will time the meal so that I eat my second meal right after I am done working out.

The meal consists of everything we ate in meal one with fewer carbohydrates and more protein from added turkey bacon.

Main Course: Protein Salad

Ingredients:

- 2 to 4 handfuls of mixed leafy greens
- 3/4 pound of ground chicken
- 3 eggs
- 6 pieces of turkey bacon
- A small handful of blueberry's
- A few mushrooms
- Walden farms zero calorie dressing

Side: Rice Cakes with Almond Butter

- 1 to 2 rice cakes
- 1 tbsp. of almond butter on each rice cake

Drink: Liver Detox Shake

- Ingredients and directions found in section 6 of this book

Main Course Instructions;

First, find a large bowl and or container. Put 2 to 4 handfuls of leafy mixed greens in the bowl.

Cook one pound of ground chicken on the stove with medium to high heat until completely done. Add your favorite seasoning in small amounts as you cook. Once the chicken is completely cooked, add it to the bowl.

Next scramble or fry 1 to 3 eggs whichever you prefer in a saucepan by first spreading one tps of grass-fed butter or olive oil in the pan on a stove with medium to high heat, adding salt and pepper if you like and once completely done, add the eggs to the bowl.

Spread a tsp of grass-fed butter or olive oil in a saucepan, place six strips of turkey bacon in the pan and cook on medium to high heat until done. Once done, add the turkey bacon strips to the salad bowl.

Finally, add your toppings blueberries and mushrooms or other vegetables to the protein salad and drizzle on as much Walden farms zero calories dressing as you like.

Side Instructions;

On a plate place 1 to 2 rice cakes. For each rice cake, you have spread one tbsp. of almond butter on it.

Estimate of Meal One

Calories: 1,043

Protein: 110g

Carbs: 27g

Fats 56g

Nine

Supplements That Will Help you get Lean and Ripped

There is a big misconception in the fitness industry that supplements are the magic behind the gains that you see the models posting when for a fact they are a very tiny piece of the puzzle.

There are only three supplements I take and by no means do you need to take them at all. You can still see amazing results without taking these supplements.

Here they are:

Carlson Cod Liver Oil, Norwegian, Lemon, 1,100 mg Omega-3s, 500 mL
https://amzn.to/2Nry6xI

NOW L-Carnitine 1000 mg, 100 Tablets
https://amzn.to/2NqR4Ve

Cruciferous Vegetable Capsules - Liver Support
https://amzn.to/2NucG2P

All these are purchasable on amazon.com. Links are provided below each supplement.

Ten

Conclusion

That's my intermittent fasting meal plan, simply two meals a day. This keeps growth hormone levels extremely high, and insulin levels low. That way it gives you the best combination of burning fat and maintaining lean muscle mass so you can get lean and ripped fast.

These are the action steps:

- ✓ Set up your eating window; 8 hour eating window, 16 hour fasting window.

- ✓ Drink plenty of water during your fasting window and if you get hungry try zero calorie drinks like sparkling water, coffee, or tea.

- ✓ Prepare and consume your meals inside the eating window you set up.

- ✓ Work out on a regular basis, it does not matter when have a routine and be consistent.

- ✓ Get plenty of sleep.

Thank you for taking the time to read my book. I did my best to make this Intermittent Fasting Meal Plan as short and to the point as possible. It's the exact intermittent fasting meal plan that I use to get lean and ripped.

If you purchased this book on Amazon and/or have watched any of my content on YouTube, thank you for the support!

Don't hesitate to DM me on any of the social media platforms that I provided at the beginning of the book, SnapChat, Instagram, or YouTube if you have any questions.

I wish you luck in your process of getting lean and ripped!

Eleven

Q & A from the YouTube Community

Joe Davis 10 months ago

Anthony Cooke I lift 4 days on. 1 off. I really want to drop body fat but still keep my muscle. When is the best time for cardio and lifting. Cardio in the morning, before first meal. Then lift before last meal?

 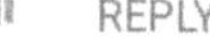 REPLY

Anthony Cooke 10 months ago

The best time is a time that works for you. It's not going to matter 'when' more than being consistent each day.

  REPLY

Joe Davis 10 months ago

Anthony Cooke thanks! I'm gonna start my first day tomorrow. Hopefully I can check in with ya. Thanks for everything

  REPLY

Anthony Cooke 10 months ago

Sounds good. You're Welcome!

  REPLY

mike varvara 1 year ago

Love the video , I have a hectic work schedule so I workout first thing in the morning . What do you suggest I can do to try IF ?

 REPLY

Hide replies ⌃

  **Anthony Cooke** 1 year ago

Working out in the morning is fine this shouldn't be a problem. You can set your eating window and fasting windows anytime you would like as long as they are consistent day to day. In this video I am just giving you an example of what times I use. Any times work.

 REPLY

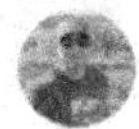
Joe Davis 10 months ago
Do you have to eat that much?

👍 👎 REPLY

Hide replies ⌃

Anthony Cooke 10 months ago
Joe Davis Nope

👍 👎 REPLY

Joe Davis 10 months ago
Anthony Cooke is there a minimum I should eat? Or in between? I like the diet, just wondering how much I should eat.

👍 👎 REPLY

Anthony Cooke 10 months ago
Joe Davis Depends on your goal. If your trying to lose fat / weight you'll need to be in a calorie deficit. If your trying to add muscle I would suggest a maintenance or slight surplus of calories.

👍 👎 REPLY

faddys1234 1 year ago
is it better to go the gym fasted and then get the fist meal 1 or 2 hours after the gym? in that way your still burning calories from body fat even after the gym.

👍 👎 REPLY

Hide replies ⌃

Anthony Cooke 1 year ago
faddys1234 As long as your following the intermittent fasting protocol when you have your first meal is up to you. Better is subjective to your situation.

👍 👎 REPLY

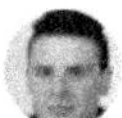
Cristian Speziale 1 year ago
This is very similar to Leangains protocol for rest days. Why do you keep carbs low and fat high also in trainign day?Did you notice more benefits?

👍 👎 REPLY

Hide replies ⌃

Anthony Cooke 1 year ago
I like higher fats. Keeps me full better, less cravings, great over all energy. I have nothing against going high on carbs. I can train more intense with higher carb intake.

👍 👎 REPLY

Taviarosie1973 1 year ago

do drink your Apple cider with a straw to protect the enamel of your teeth.!! thanks for such great info.

👍 12 👎   REPLY

Hide replies ∧

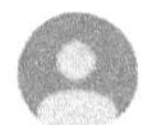

Anthony Cooke 1 year ago

I usually shoot it, or mix it with water and lemon then drink it.

👍 4 👎   REPLY

John Powers 1 year ago

Just curious; how are you able to manage/schedule all this and also maintain a meaningful job.?

👍 19 👎   REPLY

Hide replies ∧

Anthony Cooke 1 year ago

I prep my entire meals for the next day the night before, pack it in my lunch box, and off I go.

👍 42 👎   REPLY

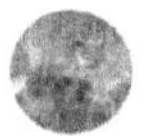

Marios Delvos 1 year ago

Hello the Apple Cider Vinegar from supermarket for food   is ok ?

👍 4 👎   REPLY

Hide replies ∧

Anthony Cooke 1 year ago

This is the brand I get "Bragg Organic Raw and Unfiltered Apple Cider Vinegar". Google that and you'll see what I am talking about.

👍 8 👎   REPLY

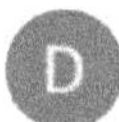

Dee Bennett 1 year ago

Is it good for women 55 and older that want to grow muscle mass.

👍 2 👎   REPLY

Hide replies ∧

Anthony Cooke 1 year ago

Intermittent fasting is a tool that can be used for either building muscle mass or burning fat and losing weight. There are going to be different aspects to it calories/macros/training wise depending on what your goal is. But yes IF will work for any age, and any fitness goal you have.

👍 1 👎   REPLY

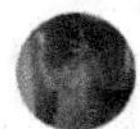

gym rabbit 1 year ago

I can't consume coffe or greentea with empty stomuch in the morning, i will feeling sick, can I eat 30 calories worth of food?

👍 4 👎   REPLY

Hide replies ⌃

Anthony Cooke 1 year ago

If you truly are intermittent fasting then that would break the protocol to eat calories during your fasting period. However that is not to say you wont see results eating 30 calories worth of food in your fasting window.

👍 3 👎   REPLY

Lina Wiklund 10 months ago

Is it better to eat two bigger meals insted of three small during the eating window? My window is 4-6 hours

👍 1 👎   REPLY

Hide replies ⌃

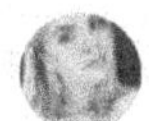

Anthony Cooke 10 months ago

Either is fine in this case. I would do whatever you can be most consistent with.

👍 1 👎   REPLY

Luis Reyes 1 year ago

I have gone from 250 to 192 in 3 months and I like the way I look I have gain muscle on the way but is there a way to lose the belly fat a lot faster or just keep doing the same thing

👍 1 👎   REPLY

Hide replies ⌃

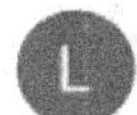

Anthony Cooke 1 year ago

Luis Reyes Its not possible to spot reduce fat, but my intuition tells me if you keep going you will lose it. Cheers from Amsterdam! 🙂 Nice work man.

👍 1 👎   REPLY

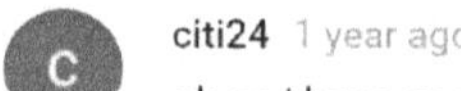

citi24 1 year ago

ok so i have my last meal 8pm yhen dont eat until 2pm. i go a full 18hrs. is that wrong? or even better? someone help

👍 1 👎   REPLY

Hide replies ⌃

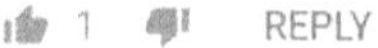

Anthony Cooke 1 year ago

Even better.

👍 3 👎   REPLY

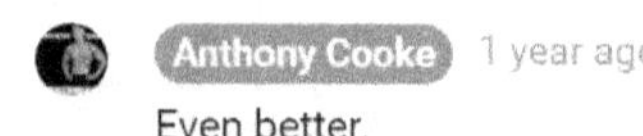

Gary Stroud 10 months ago

shouldnt be drinking coffee breaks your fast.

👍 1 👎   REPLY

Hide replies ⌃

Anthony Cooke 10 months ago

Gary Stroud If its just pure "black coffee" with nothing added it shouldn't break your fast.

👍 6 👎   REPLY

 Ado Podrinje 1 year ago

why not 6 hour window? and 18h fasting?

👍 3 👎   REPLY

Hide replies ⌃

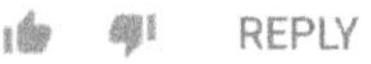

Anthony Cooke 1 year ago

Yes that would work fine as well.

👍 👎   REPLY